RICE COOKER COOKBOOK
FOR BEGINNERS

Learn How to Prepare 45+ Different Recipes with This Cookbook Along with Instructions and Guidelines to Guide You Through the Process

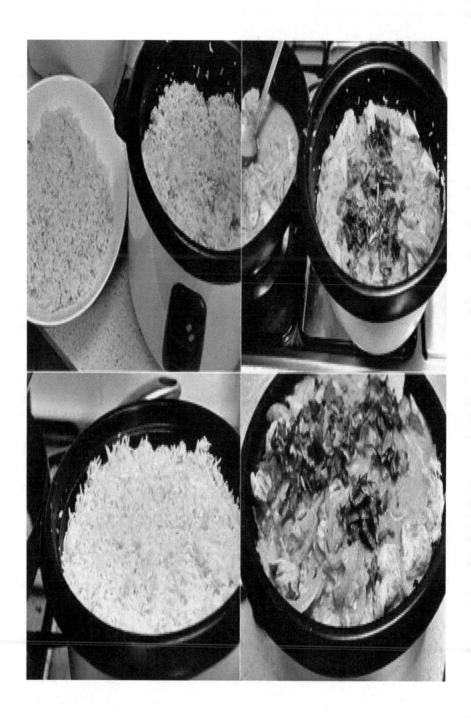

Table of Contents

INTRODUCTION

Why should we use a rice cooker?

As you may know, a rice cooker isn't the solitary piece of cooking gear you can use to cook rice. You can likewise cook rice in a burner pot or pot. Cooking rice in a pot is adequately basic – you should simply embed your ingredients, heat them to the point of boiling, turn the heat down, cover the pot, and stand by. So what's the point of messing with a rice cooker, a different gadget that appears to just have the option to do a certain something?

Since rice cookers cook rice impeccably, without fail. Indeed, even the most capable of burner rice cooks now and then end up with soft, foul rice that is crusted to the pot and difficult to clean. Furthermore, when the surface of your rice is off, the primary and textural respectability of your whole supper is in danger. The most awesome thing? With a rice cooker, you should simply stack your ingredients and press a solitary catch. There's no compelling reason to balance heat, set clocks, or even stay in a similar room as the rice while it cooks. Numerous advanced rice cookers have highlights that permit you to plan rice cooking for later in the day, keep the rice warm when it's finished cooking, steam different ingredients like vegetables, and that's only the tip of the iceberg.

Rice cooker meals for beginners

45+ recipes

1.   Easy Vegetable Biryani

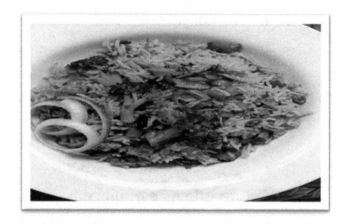

Planning time: 10 mins

Cook time: 30 mins

Complete time: 40 mins

Serves: 4

1) Fixings

    a. 1 cup of basmati or any since a long time ago grained rice

b. 2 cups of blended vegetables, hacked (I use what I have close by - broccoli, carrots, beans, cauliflower, peas, corn, infant corn, capsicum, and so on)

c. 2 tsp. of biryani masala (or 3 cloves, 3 cardamom, 1" piece cinnamon, 1 star anise)

d. 1 fistful of mint leaves

e. 1 little bundle of coriander leaves (cilantro)

f. ½ tsp. of turmeric powder

g. ½ tsp. of cumin seeds

h. 1 tsp. of coriander powder

i. 2-3 green chilies, minced

j. 1 tsp. of red stew powder (change in accordance with taste)

k. 2 enormous onions, cut

l. ½ cup of curd (discretionary)

m. 1 tbsp. of ghee

n. A few cashew nuts or almonds (discretionary)

o. 1 tsp. of ginger garlic glue

Technique

1. Wash the rice and absorb it some water while you go about with the remainder of the arrangements.

2. Warmth the ghee in a wide dish and meal the nuts (if utilizing) Drain and add the cut onions and meal until brilliant earthy colored.

3. Put to its side portion and add ginger garlic glue. Sauté until fragrant.

4. Then, add the green chilies, stew powder, turmeric, coriander powder, cumin, and some salt. Sauté until the flavors are cooked – around 1 moment.

5. Finish off with the hacked vegetables and blend well. Add the biryani masala and the slashed mint and coriander leaves (see notes on the best way to utilize entire flavors).

6. Move this to your rice cooker dish and add around 2 cups water and the curd – the estimations will change as per rice cooker utilized – and the doused rice. (See notes for pressure cooker biryani strategy).

7. At the point when the rice is done, open quickly and give it a decent mix through when still hot. Add the saved simmered nuts and onions.

8. Enhancement with more coriander leaves and sprinkle some lemon juice whenever wanted.

9. Present with papad or chips and a pleasant cooling raita.

2. Easy Rice Cooker Chicken Curry

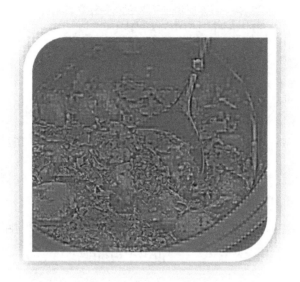

Prepared IN: 30mins

SERVES: 4

Fixings

1) 2 tablespoons oil

2) 1 cup cleaved onion

3) 1 tablespoon minced garlic

4) 2 tablespoons curry powder

5) 2 cups water

6) 1 (8 ounce) would tomato be able to sauce

7) 1 (8 ounce) bundle zatarain's jambalaya blend

8) 1 lb. boneless skinless chicken bosom, cut into 1-inch solid shapes

9) 1/2 cup brilliant raisin

10)   3/4 cup plain yogurt

11)   1/3 cup cleaved cashews

Headings

1.   Hit Cook and spot oil in container at that point Add onion and garlic; cook and mix 5 minutes or until onion is delicate. Add curry powder; cook and mix 2 minutes.

2.   Add water, pureed tomatoes, and Jambalaya Mix chicken and raisins blend well.

3.   Close Lid and hit COOK after cooker exchanged over to Warm mood killer the Rice cooker and mix in yogurt.

4.   Let stand 5 minutes. Sprinkle with cashews.

3. Rice Cooker Quinoa Mushroom Pilaf

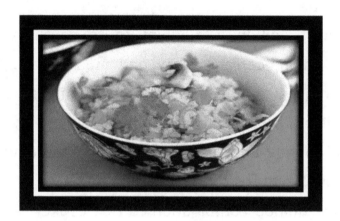

Time: 45 minutes

Serving: 4

Fixings

1) 1 cup white quinoa, absorbed water for 15 minutes, at that point flushed altogether, and depleted

2) 1 Tbs. olive oil

3) 1 clove garlic, minced

4) 1/2 cup onion, finely cleaved

5) 1/2 cup carrot, finely cleaved

6) 1/2 cup celery, finely cleaved

7) 1 cup mushrooms, cut

8) 1/2 tsp. turmeric

9) 1/2 cup red ringer pepper, finely hacked

10) 1 3/4 cup low sodium vegetable or chicken stock

Technique

1. Warmth oil in a medium sauté container. Add garlic, onion, carrot, celery and mushrooms. Sauté until onions are mollified and mushrooms are daintily carmelized, around 3 to 4 minutes.

2. Add quinoa and turmeric and keep sautéing for 2 additional minutes to toast quinoa.

3. Move quinoa combination to rice cooker. Add red chime pepper and stock.

4. Cook on "white rice" setting.

4. Rice Cooker Frittata with Summer Vegetables

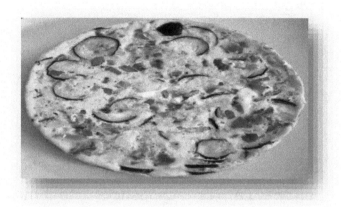

Time: 35 minutes

Makes 2 to 4 servings

Fixings

1) The vegetables:

   a. 1 entire garlic clove, stripped

   b. 1 little red or yellow pepper, cut into little dice

   c. 1 little potato, stripped and finely julienned

   d. 1 little zucchini, cut into slender rounds

   e. salt and pepper

   f. 1 Tbs. olive oil

2) The egg combination: 6 huge eggs 2 Tbs. ground cheddar of any sort (discretionary) salt and pepper 1 Tbs. olive oil

3) Hardware required:
   a. Rice cooker
   b. Frying skillet
   c. Burner or oven (see Notes for what to do in the event that you don't have a burner or oven)
   d. chopsticks or fork to blend the eggs
   e. spatula or chopsticks to mix the vegetables around

Technique

1.   Heat up the griddle with 1 tablespoon of olive oil. Add the garlic clove, and let the oil heat up until the garlic is daintily earthy colored. Dispose of the garlic clove.

2.   Add the vegetables. The key with the vegetables is to cut them up as little and meagerly is you can, so they cook quickly. Season with salt and pepper. Put in a safe spot.

3.   Put 1 tablespoon of olive oil in the rice cooker bowl. Spread it around the base and around 2 inches/5 cm up the sides, utilizing a paper towel. Add the eggs, ground cheddar, salt and pepper, and beat the eggs in the bowl (take care not to start to expose what's underneath in case you're utilizing a metal fork for this). Add the vegetables and disseminate them equitably in the egg combination.

4.   Put the bowl in the rice cooker and switch on, utilizing the standard rice setting. At the point when the cooking cycle completes, the frittata is finished! Here's what it looks like straight out of the cooker:

5.   Let cool totally prior to cutting into wedges and getting together for a bento.

6.   Optionally add a little ketchup or pureed tomatoes prior to eating.

5. Chicken & Daikon Soup Recipe

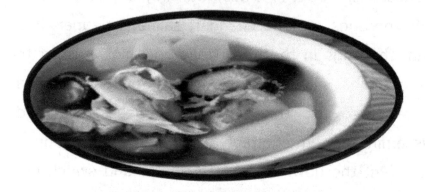

Serves: 2-3

Planning Time: 10 mins

Cook Time: 3 hrs.

Fixings:

1) 500g chicken skin eliminated and cleaved to more modest pieces(I utilize 3 huge chicken drumsticks, you can likewise utilize half chicken or chicken thighs)

2) 1 liter of water

3) 5 cuts of ginger

4) 1 daikon (white radish/) about 300g, stripped and slice to huge pieces

5) 8 shiitake mushrooms stems eliminated

6) 1 tbsp. wolfberries absorbed water until puffy; depleted

7) 3 dried scallops

8) salt to taste

9) Apparatuses Needed

10) A essential "keep warm/cook" electronic rice cooker

Bearings:

1. Add water to the rice cooker pot, set to "Cook". At the point when the water bubbles, add chicken in the rice cooker for 5-8 minutes with the rice cooker covered and dispose of the primary difference in cooking fluid. Put to the side whitened chicken pieces.

2. Add 1 liter of water to the rice cooker pot, cover and set to 'Cook'.

3. When the water bubbles, add chicken, daikon, mushrooms, dried scallops and ginger. Cover the rice cooker and get back to a bubble. I leave the soup in the 'Cook' mode for around 45 minutes.

4. Switch the rice cooker to 'Warm' and permit to stew for in any event another 1-2 hours.

5. 15 to 30 minutes prior to serving the soup, add the splashed wolfberries. Add salt to taste.

6. Steamed Salmon with Brown Rice

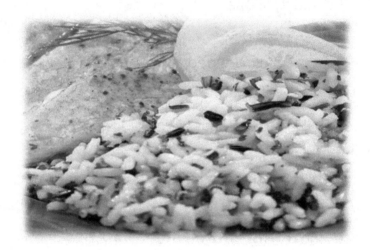

Time: 45 minutes

Serving 3/4

Fixings

1) 2 salmon filets (wild Alaskan, 3–4 ounces/85–113 g each)

2) 2 tsp. (10 ml) ground ginger

3) 3 tbsp. (45 ml) low-sodium soy sauce

4) 1 garlic clove, minced

5) 2 tsp. (10 ml) dim earthy colored sugar

6) 1/2 tsp. (2.5 ml) bean stew drops

7) 1 green onion or shallot, cut

8) Brown rice (uncooked)

9) Salt and pepper, to taste

Headings

1. Spot liner container on plate (to get any drippings).

2. Blend ginger, soy sauce, garlic, dull earthy colored sugar, and bean stew pieces.

3. Rub fish filets with blend and spot in cooler to marinate for roughly 30 minutes.

4. Measure earthy colored rice as indicated by wanted servings/bundle bearings. Fill cooking pot to relating water line (see Rice Chart for extra data). Chicken or vegetable stock/stock may likewise be filling in for water.

5. Set Simplicity Cooker: Whole Grain—after roughly 30–35 minutes, lift cover and add liner bushel with salmon filets.

6. Cook an extra 8–10 minutes or until salmon pieces effectively with a fork.

7. Serve salmon over rice and sprinkle with cut green onion.

7.   Balsamic Dijon Chicken with Farro & Mushrooms

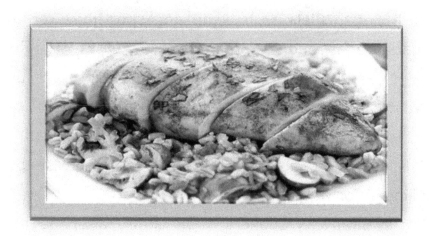

SERVINGS: 4

Planning TIME: 20 min

COOK TIME: 60 min

Length: 80 min

Fixings

1) 4 5-oz boneless, skinless chicken bosoms

2) 1 tsp. olive oil

3) 2 shallots, minced

4) 8 oz. cremini mushrooms, quartered

5) 1 cup farro

6) 1 1/2 cups low-sodium vegetable stock

7) 1/4 cup minced new parsley

8) Marinade

9) 1/3 cup balsamic vinegar

10)   1 tsp. extra-virgin olive oil

11)   1 tbsp. Dijon mustard

12)   Pinch every ocean salt and ground dark pepper

- Preparation

1. Prepare marinade: In a bowl or zip-top plastic sack, join all marinade fixings. Add chicken, going to guarantee that bosoms are totally covered with marinade. Cover bowl with saran wrap or seal sack and refrigerate until required.

2. Set your rice cooker to the "ordinary" setting. Spot 1 tsp. oil in rice cooker bowl. Add shallots, mixing to cover, at that point close or cover with top. Cook for around 5 minutes, mixing once in a while, until shallots have mellowed. Add mushrooms and cook for 8 additional minutes, covered and mixing once in a while, until mushrooms are delicate and have delivered water. Mix in farro and cook, revealed and blending sometimes, for 3 minutes.

3.   Stir in stock. Spot chicken, disposing of extra marinade, on top of farro blend. Close or cover with top and reset rice cooker to "standard" setting. The program should require around 60 minutes, contingent upon the rice cooker. Chicken is done when its interior temperature arrives at 165°F.

4.   To serve, place 3/4 cup farro-mushroom combination on each plate and top with 1 chicken bosom.

5.   Sprinkle with parsley, separating equitably.

8. Rice Cooker Super Cheesy Polenta

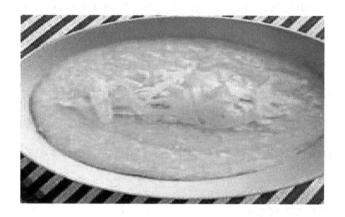

Prep: 10 mins

Cook: 30 mins

Absolute: 40 mins

Servings: 4

Fixings

1) 2 tablespoons spread

2) ½ onion, hacked

3) 1 clove garlic, minced

4) 1 cup chicken stock

5) 1 cup milk

6) ½ cup polenta

7) ¼ teaspoon salt, or more to taste

8) 2 ounces destroyed cheddar

9) 2 ounces destroyed Parmesan cheddar

10)   ¼ teaspoon newly ground dark pepper

Bearings

1. Spot spread, onion, and garlic in rice cooker; close cover and turn on cooker. Cook until onion is delicate and clear, blending sporadically, 10 to 15 minutes. Add chicken stock, milk, polenta, and salt.

2. Cover and cook on full cycle, mixing sometimes, until polenta has retained the fluid, around 20 minutes.

3. Add cheddar, Parmesan cheddar, and dark pepper; mix until cheddar is liquefied.

9.   Rice Cooker Rice Pudding

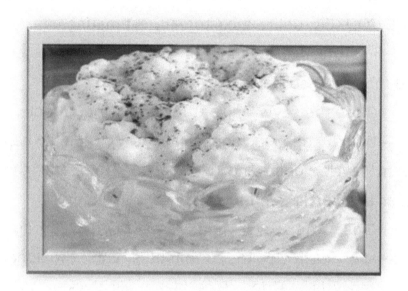

Planning Time: 10 mins

Cook Time: 2 hrs. 50 mins

Refrigerate Time: 1 hr.

Absolute Time: 4 hrs.

Servings: 4 servings

Fixings

1) ⅔ c rice long grain or short grain, uncooked

2) 4 c milk

3) ⅓ c sugar

4) 1 tsp. vanilla concentrate

Directions

1.   DO NOT USE THE CUP THAT COMES WITH THE RICE COOKER, utilize a customary estimating cup!

2.   Put the rice and milk in the rice cooker bowl and mix to consolidate.

3.   Close the cover and set for the Porridge cycle.

4.   When the machine changes to the "Keep Warm" cycle, open the rice cooker, and add the sugar and vanilla, and mix until consolidated.

5.   Close the cover and reset briefly Porridge cycle. Mix each 15 to 20 minutes until the ideal consistency is reached. Rice blend will thicken as it cools. In the event that it comes out too thick, simply add more milk.

6.   Serve warm or let cool somewhat and refrigerate for at any rate 60 minutes.

7.   When cold, cover with saran wrap and store for as long as 4 days.

10. Rice Cooker Ginger Chicken and Rice

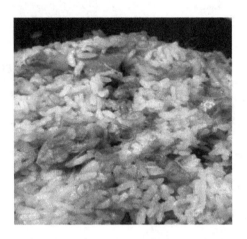

Dynamic: 15 mins

Total: 1 hr.

Servings: 4

Fixings

1) 1 enormous chicken bouillon 3D shape, ideally all-regular

2) 3/4 cup boiling water

3) 1 cup jasmine rice

4) 1/4 pounds skinless, boneless chicken thighs, cut into 1-inch blocks

5) One 2-inch piece of new ginger, stripped and cut into matchsticks

6) 3 pressed cups child spinach

7) 1 cup unsweetened coconut milk

8) Kosher salt

Headings

1. In a little bowl, disintegrate the bouillon 3D shape in the hot water. In a rice cooker, join the rice with the chicken and ginger.

2. Mastermind the spinach on top. Pour the coconut milk and bouillon stock into the cooker and season softly with salt.

3. Turn the cooker on; the dish ought to be done in around 40 minutes (when the cooker turns itself off). Let represent 5 minutes.

4. Cushion the rice with a fork, spoon into bowls and serve.

11. Char Siu (Chinese Style Roast Pork) Made in a Rice Cooker

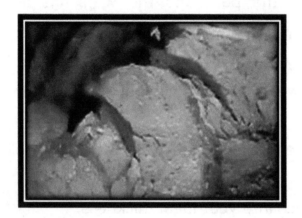

Time: 55 minutes

Serving: 2

Fixings

1.   350 grams Pork for making broil pork (flimsy square)

2.   40 ml ★ Soy sauce

3.   100 ml ★Sake

4.   100 ml Mirin

5.   50 ml ★ Water

6.   1 piece/clove each ★ Ginger and garlic

Steps

1.   Make the slim square of pork prepared.

2.   Brown the outside of the pork in a skillet. You don't have to cook it through, you simply need to brown it.

3.   Put the pork and the ★ fixings in the rice cooker and switch it on. On the off chance that you have any extra pieces of green onion or leek and other sweet-smelling vegetables, put those in as well.

4.   The pork is done when the rice cooker turns off.

5.   Slice into your ideal thickness.

12. Cook Eggs in a Rice Cooker

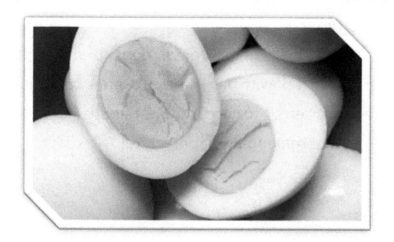

Planning Time: 1 moment

Cook Time: 20 minutes

Chilling time: 1 moment

All out Time: 21 minutes

Fixings

1) eggs

2) 1 - 1 ½ cups water around

3) Bowl of ice water (can be two or three minutes before eggs are finished cooking)

Directions

1.   Add water to rice pot and set into cooker.

2.   Place eggs in liner plate and set in rice pot. Close cooker top.

3.   Set rice cooker to COOK and begin the cooker and clock simultaneously. (See Notes underneath for cooking times.)

4.   Once clock rings, move eggs promptly to a bowl loaded up with ice water to stop the cooking interaction. Let sit for around 1-2 minutes.

5.   Start breaking and appreciate!

13. Rice Cooker Sausage Jambalaya

Time: 55 minutes

Servings: 3/4

Fixings

1) 1/2 lb. smoked wiener, meagerly cut
2) 1/2 can French onion soup (around a 1/2 cup)
3) 1/2 cup water
4) 1 can Rotel (gentle) or diced tomatoes, undrained
5) 1 can black-eyed peas, undrained
6) 1 1/2 cups uncooked rice*
7) *If utilizing the rice cooker estimating cup, utilize 2 of those cups for the rice since they are really 3/4 cup.

Directions

1.　Mix all fixings in rice cooker.

2.　Start the rice cooker.

3.　Once it completes, permit it to set for 5 minutes. (Try not to lift the top).

4.　Turn the rice cooker back on once more. It will cook for a more limited cycle this time. Allow it to set for 10 minutes after it goes off.

5.　Stir and check rice to ensure it is finished.

6.　If not, add somewhat more water (around 2 tbsp.), mix, and set it to cook once more.

14. Rice Cooker Chinese Sticky Rice

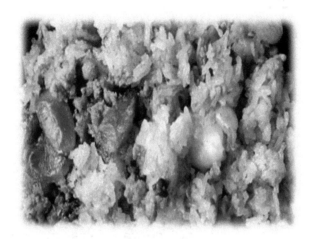

Planning Time: 20 minutes

Cook Time: 25 minutes

Splashing time: 2 hours

Complete Time: 45 minutes

Makes: servings 10

Fixings

1) 2 cups Thai glutinous rice (see note underneath)

2) ½ lb. (225g) ground pork

3) ¼ lb. (115g) shrimp, deveined and shells and tails eliminated (around 12 medium-sized)

4) 2 Chinese hotdogs

5) 2-3 medium estimated dried shiitake mushrooms

6) 1 ¼ cups water

7) Sauce:

8) 3 tablespoons shellfish sauce

9) 1 tablespoons soy sauce (tamari for without gluten)

10)   1 teaspoon ground ginger

11)   1 clove garlic, minced or ground

12)   ½ teaspoon custard starch (cornstarch OK)

13)   ½ teaspoon sesame oil

14)   ¼ teaspoon white pepper

Directions

Splashing:

1.   Place dried mushrooms in a bowl with heated water and let splash for in any event 2 hours until relaxed. (See note beneath)

2.   Run virus water through the rice in a sifter. Mix the rice with your hand to wash and flush it well until the water is generally running clear.

3.   Soak the rice in a bowl of water for in any event 2 hours.

At the point when prepared to cook:

1. Combine the 3 tablespoons shellfish sauce, 1 tablespoon soy sauce (or tamari), 1 teaspoon ground ginger, minced garlic clove, ½ teaspoon custard starch, ½ teaspoon sesame oil, and ¼ teaspoon white pepper in a bowl and blend well to make the sauce. Put in a safe spot.

2. Drain the rice through a colander, disposing of the water.

3. Remove mushrooms from splashing fluid and delicately crush out a portion of the water. Cut of and dispose of intense stems. Cut mushroom covers into cuts or lumps.

4. Slice Chinese hotdogs into plates.

5. Heat a skillet over medium warmth. Add Chinese hotdog and ground pork and cook until pork is for the most part cooked through.

6. Add mushrooms and sauce to the dish and mix. Warmth through.

7. Add shrimp and cook until simply beginning to become pink and eliminate from heat.

8. Transfer Chinese frankfurter blend to the rice cooker pot and level out.

9. Add depleted rice on top and level out.

10. Add 1 ¼ cups water to the rice cooker.

11.   Cook until rice cooker button pops, or for around 25 minutes. Let sit for another 5-10 minutes. Rice ought to be totally cooked and marginally clear.

12.   Fluff rice with chopsticks, mixing great to blend the rice and filling fixings.

13.   Garnish with hacked green onions, whenever wanted.

15. Teriyaki Pulled Chicken

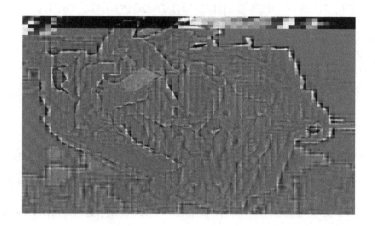

Planning Time: 15 minutes

Cook Time: 6 hours

All out Time: 6 hours 15 minutes

Fixings

1) 4 skinless, boneless chicken bosoms

2) 2 skinless, boneless chicken thighs

3) ¼ cup tamari (soy sauce if not GF)

4) ¼ cup nectar

5) 2 cloves garlic minced

6) 2 tbsp. ginger minced

7) 1 tbsp. rice vinegar

8) ¼ tsp. white pepper

9) 1 tbsp. custard starch (or cornstarch)

10)   2 tbsp. water

Guidelines

1.   Combine soy sauce, nectar, garlic, ginger, rice vinegar, and white pepper in a bowl and blend well.

2.   Combine chicken pieces and marinade in lethargic cooker pot.

3.   Cook on high for 4-6 hours; low for 6-8 hours.

4.   Remove chicken and shred.

5.   Pour fluid from moderate cooker into an enormous pan or skillet over medium-low warmth.

6.   Mix custard flour and water into a slurry and mix into the sauce to thicken.

7.   Add pulled chicken to the pan and blend in with the thickened sauce.

8.   Serve right away.

16. Red Beans and Rice

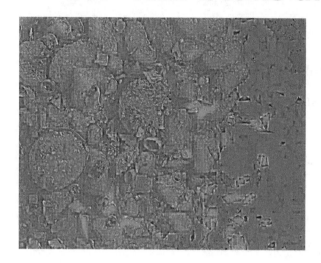

Time: 35 minutes

Servings: 2/3

Fixings:

1) 1 cup white rice

2) 1¼ cups water

3) 1½ teaspoons ground cumin

4) 2 teaspoons legitimate salt

5) 3 teaspoons stew powder

6) 1½ teaspoons garlic powder

7) ¾ teaspoon smoked paprika

8) 1 green chime pepper, finely diced

9) 1 yellow onion, finely diced

10)   ½ pound ham, finely diced

11)   1 can red kidney beans, depleted and flushed

Bearings:

1. In a rice cooker, consolidate rice, water, flavors, chime pepper, and onion. Start cooker.

2. Following 10 minutes, mix in ham. Permit cooker to complete its cycle.

3. Mix in kidney beans and close cover.

4. Leave on warm 5 to 10 minutes until beans are warmed through prior to serving.

17. Mac and Cheese

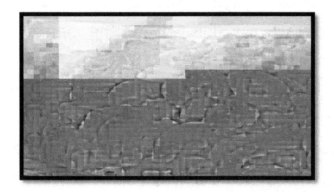

Time: 20 minutes

Serving: 3

Fixings:

1) 2 cups elbow macaroni

2) 1 teaspoon legitimate salt

3) 1 (12-ounce) can dissipated milk

4) ¾ cup destroyed cheddar

5) ¾ cup cubed handled cheddar item

6) ½ teaspoon mustard powder

7) ½ teaspoon newly ground dark pepper

Bearings:

1. Consolidate the macaroni, salt, and 2 cups water in a rice cooker.

2. Set the rice cooker on the standard white rice cycle and cook for 30 minutes, or until the cooking cycle is practically finished and the majority of the water is assimilated.

3. Mix in the milk, cheddar, handled cheddar item, mustard, and dark pepper.

4. Close the cover, turn the cooker to the warm setting, and let cook, mixing incidentally so the base doesn't consume.

5. until the cheddar is dissolved and the milk is all around consolidated, around 10 minutes.

18. Rice Cooker Chicken Chili

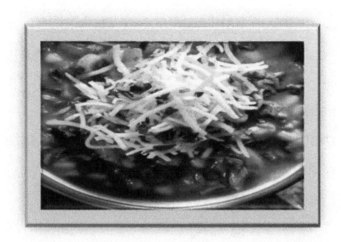

Time: 35 minutes

Servings: 4

Fixings:

1) 1 pound ground chicken
2) 1 can dark beans
3) 1 can kidney beans
4) 1 tablespoon bean stew powder
5) 1 tablespoon tomato glue
6) 1 cup pureed tomatoes
7) ½ parcel of your decision of bean stew preparing
8) 2 teaspoon dried oregano

9) Salt and pepper to taste

Headings:

1. Spot crude ground chicken in rice cooker, turn it on, and let it run until completely cooked.

2. When carmelized and completely cooked through, channel overabundance fat. Add beans, pureed tomatoes, tomato glue, and mix.

3. At that point, include all flavors and let stew for another full cycle on the rice cooker.

19. Mushroom Risotto

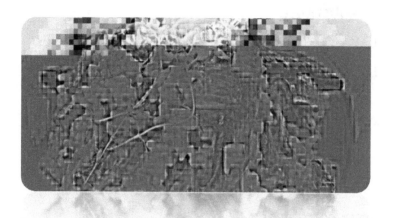

Time: 30 minutes

Serving: 3

Fixings:

1) ½ cup minced white onion
2) 3 cloves minced garlic
3) 1 tablespoon olive oil
4) 4 ounces mushrooms, slashed or broken into little pieces
5) 1 teaspoon salt
6) 1 teaspoon thyme
7) ½ cup dry white wine, room temperature
8) 3 cups vegetable stock, room temperature
9) 1 cup Arborio rice
10)   ¼ cup lemon juice

11) 2 cups new spinach

12) 1 tablespoon vegetarian spread substitute

13) 1½ tablespoons wholesome yeast

14) Black pepper, to taste

Headings:

1. Turn your rice cooker on, however leave the cover open Add the oil to the rice cooker and let it heat while you prep the fixings Add the onions and garlic, and mix to relax.

2. Mix in the mushrooms, salt, and thyme. Add the wine and vegetable stock, mix well. Add the rice, mix well once more. Close the rice cooker top and restart the cooking clock. Allow the rice to cook for the endorsed cycle, when complete, mix well.

3. Move into a serving bowl and mix in: lemon juice, spinach, veggie lover spread substitute, healthful yeast, and dark pepper.

4. Mix until the veggie lover margarine substitute totally melts and all fixings are blended together well.

5. Serve warm, finished off with slashed spinach, whenever wanted.

20. Chicken and Chinese Sausage Rice

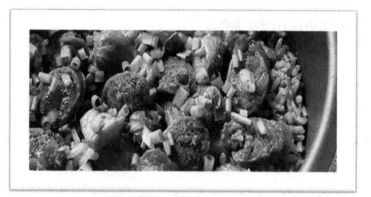

Time: 45 minutes

Serving: 3/4

Fixings

1) 3 cups uncooked Jasmine rice (utilize the cup from rice cooker)

2) 600 ml water (as much depending on the situation by the rice cooker)

3) 300 gr boneless chicken thigh, cubed

4) 3 lap cheong (Chinese frankfurter), cut

5) 5 garlic cloves, minced

6) 2 cm ginger, minced

7) 2 tbsp. shellfish sauce

8) 2-3 tbsp. light soy sauce (to taste)

9) Ground white pepper to taste

10) 2 tsp. sesame oil

11) Green onion, cut for embellish

12) Marination for chicken :

13) 1 tsp. light soy sauce

14) Ground white pepper

Steps

1. Marinate the chicken briefly while setting up the rice.

2. Rinse the rice until the water clear at that point channels it.

3. Push the "COOK" catch of rice cooker.

4. Heat sesame oil into rice cooker bowl.

5. Add minced garlic and ginger.

6. Sauté until scent.

7. Add the rice, water, soy sauce, clam sauce and pepper. Mix it well.

8. Arrange the chicken and wiener on top of the rice.

9. Close the top of the rice cooker. Ensure the catch "COOK" is on.

10. After the rice is cooked, sprinkle with green onion.

21. Refried beans

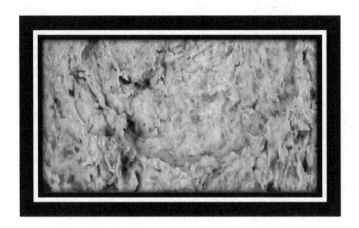

Time: 30 minutes

Serving: 4

Fixings

1) 2 C dry pinto beans

2) Quartered onion

3) clove Garlic

4) leaf Bay

5) Water or chicken stock

6) Small can hacked jalapeños or new pepper of decision

7) 3 oz. Cream cheddar

8) Salt

9) Pepper

10)   Cumin

11)   Chili powder

Steps

1.   Soak 2 C beans for the time being in rice cooker covered with water

2.   Drain and wash beans and rice cooker.

3.   Add back to rice cooker cover with chicken stock or water, a narrows leaf, quarter of an onion, a garlic clove and cook through 2 white rice cycles.

4.   Remove inlet leaf onion and garlic and dispose of. Cycle in two bunches in blender with a little water or chicken stock. Make one smooth bunch and one stout for various surfaces at that point overlay the two together.

5.   If you are utilizing a new pepper cleave up and sauté in a little oil in a skillet until delicate.

6.   Add beans, canned jalapeno, and 3oz cream cheddar in skillet season with salt pepper stew powder and cumin to taste. Sauté until cream cheddar very much consolidated.

7.   Remove from warmth and serve, ideally with cheddar.

22. Easy Homemade Mango Sticky Rice

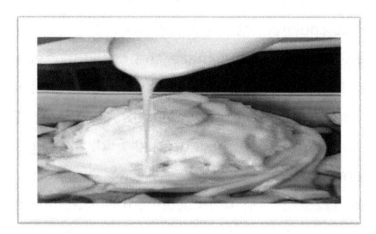

Time: 30 minutes

Serving: 4

Fixings

1) 1 cup glutinous rice (Sticky rice) wash and channel well

2) 1 cup water

3) 1 would coconut be able to drain

4) 1/2 cup sugar

5) 1/8 tsp. salt

6) 1-2 tbsp. cornstarch

7) 2-3 tsp. water

8) Fresh mango

Steps

1.   Put the glutinous rice into the rice cooker. Add 1 cup water. Ensure the rice cover with the water.

2.   Closed the rice cooker and change to cook. After it quits cooking, let it stay on "warm"

3.   Then you can begin make the coconut cream sauce. Add the coconut milk into bowl (microwave safe), add sugar, and salt. Microwave it for 2 moments. Take off then mixing great until the sugar disintegrates.

4.   Pour 1/2 - 1 cup the coconut milk blend into rice cooker. Mix rapidly to blend. At that point switch the rice cooker on "cook" once more. At the point when it stops, and the rice is done (I like to keep it warm)

5.   Now in a little bowl join he cornstarch and water. At that point fill coconut milk. Take it to the microwave. Also, microwave like clockwork, eliminate and mix until the blend turns out to be somewhat thick (around 2 minutes)

6.   To serve, move the tacky rice into serving plate or bowl.

7.   Peel and cut the mango as you want place the cut mango on the top or side of the rice.

8.   Then pour not many spoonful of the coconut cream sauce over the rice. Appreciate! Glad Cooking.

23. Rice cooker pangasius fish with capsicums

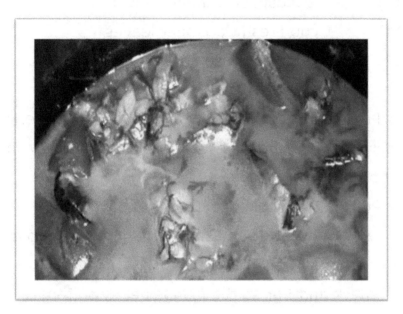

Time: 45 minutes

8-10 servings

Fixings

1) 5-7 little onion slashed

2) chili powder(as per taste)

3) 1-1.5 teaspoon turmeric powder

4) 2 teaspoon coriander powder

5) 4-5 tablespoons oil

6) Salt according to taste (1.5-2 tablespoons)

7) Water

8) 2-3 cup Capsicums

9) 8-10 piece Pangasius fish

10) 1-2 teaspoon cumin seeds powder

11) 1 cup Fresh Coriander leaves

12) You can likewise add tomatoes

Steps

1. Put Onion, bean stew powder, turmeric powder, coriander powder, oil, salt, one and half cup water together.

2. Put the rice cooker to Cook

3. Check and Stir so it doesn't adhere at bottom. Put Cooker to warm around 20 min

4. Check and Stir so the fixings nearly softens

5. At 25 min put cooker to Cook. Add capsicums

6. Add water. Carry the combination to bubble. Mix the blend.

7. Add fish and coriander leaves and Cumin seed powder

8. After 5 min mix delicately 1-2 times. Carry the pot to bubble and stand by till the water is lesser.

9. After 10 min taste to add salt if important

10. Check the level of the curry if agreeable. Put cooker to warm and serve.

24. Pork Belly made by Rice Cooker

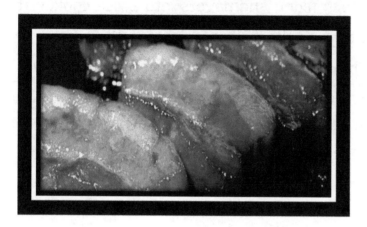

Time: 45 minutes

Serving: 2

Fixings

1) 600 g Pork paunch

2) 3 Green onion

3) 10 g Sliced Ginger

4) 5 pieces Garlic

5) (Seasoning)

6) 100 cc Water

7) 4 tbsp. Soy sauce

8) 3 tbsp. Sake

9) 3 tbsp. Mirin

10)   1.5 tbsp. Sugar

Steps

1.　Cut the pork midsection into enormous pieces. Sear it until light sautéed.

2.　Put each fixing and flavors into a rice cooker at that point turn on the switch for cooking☆

3.　30 minutes after the fact, turn the meat over and leave it for 30 minutes once more.

4.　Turn the rice cooker off then prepared for serve.

25. Red Lentil Turnip Curry (Rice Cooker Version)

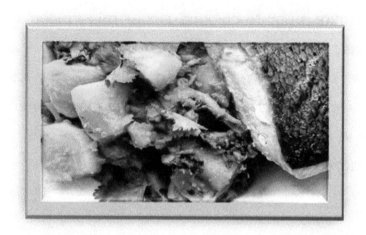

Time: 35 minutes

Serving: 4

Fixings

1) 3 enormous turnips

2) 1/2 cup red lentils

3) 1 cup dashi stock (or vegetable stock)

4) 2 tsp. curry powder

5) 1 cup mushrooms (any sort)

6) 1 cup generally cleaved Bok choy/spinach

7) Parsley

8) Lemon cuts (Optional)

Steps

1.   Peel, Dice and cleave turnips

2.   Place red lentils, stock, curry powder, turnips, mushrooms (in a specific order) in rice cooker. Cook in typical rice mode

3.   10 mins prior to cooking closes mix in cleaved parsley and Bok choy.

4.   We served it with seared salmon. You can obviously go absolutely veggie lover and increment the sum lentils in the curry.

5.   Freezes well and get scrumptious!

26. Rice Cooker Chicken

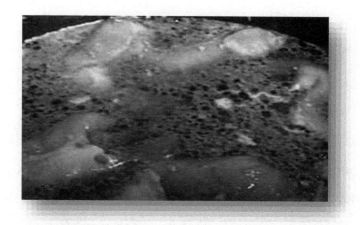

Prep: 10 mins

Cook: 45 mins

Extra: 1 hr.

All out: 1 hr. 55 mins

Servings: 4

Unique formula yields 4 servings

Fixing

1) ½ cup soy sauce

2) 6 cloves garlic, crushed

3) 4 cuts new ginger root, coarsely slashed

4) 1 teaspoon monosodium glutamate (like Ac'cent®) (Optional)

5) 1 teaspoon salt

6) ½ teaspoon ground dark pepper

7) ½ teaspoon sesame seed oil

8) 4 boneless chicken thighs

9) 1 ½ teaspoons cornstarch

10) 1 cup water, or depending on the situation - separated

Bearings

1. Spot the soy sauce, garlic, ginger, monosodium glutamate (if utilizing), salt, pepper, and sesame oil into an enormous resealable plastic pack and press the sack with your fingers to blend the fixings and break up the salt.

2. Add the chicken thighs to the marinade and crush the sack again to cover the chicken. Extract however much air as could be expected from the sack and zip the pack shut. Refrigerate for 60 minutes.

3. Blend the cornstarch and 2 tablespoons of water in a little bowl until smooth. Pour the marinade from the plastic pack into a programmable electric rice cooker and blend in the cornstarch combination until completely joined.

4. Spot the chicken thighs into the sauce. Add barely sufficient water to scarcely cover the chicken and mix.

5. Close the top of the cooker, set the cooker for the normal rice setting, and press the beginning catch. At the point when steam starts emerging from the highest point of the cooker (after around 20 minutes), set the cooker's clock for 10 minutes.

6. At the point when the clock goes off, uncover and mix the chicken. Set clock and cook for an additional 10 minutes; change the cooker to the keep-warm setting. Permit chicken to rest in the save warm setting for 20 minutes prior to serving.

27. Rice cooker chicken and bacon risotto

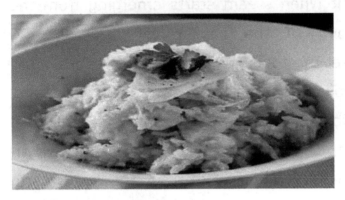

Time: 35 minutes

Serving: 4

Fixings

1) 30 g spread

2) 2 garlic cloves, squashed

3) 1 medium earthy colored onion, diced

4) 4 center bacon rashers, diced

5) 1 1/2 cups Arborio rice

6) 2 tbsp. chicken stock powder

7) 3 cups bubbling water

8) 1 twofold chicken bosom filet, diced

9) 1 cup parmesan cheddar, ground

10)   parsley (to serve)

Strategy

1. Set the rice cooker to cook position and spot spread, garlic, onion and bacon into the bowl. Fry until the onion is clear.

2. Add the rice and cook for 2-3 minutes guaranteeing that the grains are covered in the margarine. Add the stock powder, bubbling water and chicken. Mix to join, ensuring the cook button is still down.

3. Cook for roughly 15-20 minutes or until the rice is cooked yet at the same time has a firm nibble. On the off chance that it is a little dry simply add a couple of tablespoons of water and mix.

4. Mix in parmesan cheddar, embellish with parsley and serve.

28. Rice Cooker Chicken Bog

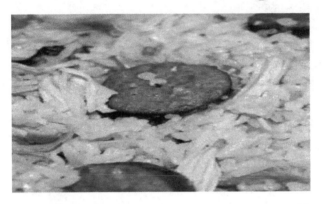

Prepared IN: 1hr 30mins

SERVES: 10

Fixings

1) 2 lbs. chicken thighs, skin on

2) 2 lbs. smoked hotdog, sliced 1/2-inch thick

3) 2 cuts pepper bacon, thick cut

4) 1 cup onion, hacked

5) 2 tablespoons spread

6) 2 teaspoons preparing salt, Lawry's

7) 1 teaspoon garlic powder

8) 1 teaspoon onion powder

9) 1 1/2 teaspoons dark pepper

10)   1/4 teaspoon cayenne pepper, overlook in the event that you don't need the warmth

11)   6 cups chicken stock

12)   3 cups crude white rice

Bearings

1.   In a huge pot over medium warmth cook the bacon until it is fresh. Eliminate and put to the side to cool. Disintegrate once cooled.

2.   Add the spread to the bacon oil and earthy colored the sausage.

3.   Add the onions and cook until they start to brown.

4.   Place the chicken thighs in the pot and add the chicken stock.

5.   Add the disintegrated bacon, season salt, garlic powder, onion powder, dark pepper and cayenne in the event that you are utilizing it.

6.   Bring the pot to a bubble and afterward put on low warmth to cook the chicken, around 30-40 minutes.

7.   Cut off the warmth and eliminate the chicken thighs. Allow them to cool, dispose of the skins and take the meat out the bones. Return the chicken meat to the pot.

8.   Place the 3 cups of rice in your rice cooker and dump in the whole substance of the pot.

9.   Push the "cook" button on your rice cooker - toward the finish of the cycle you will have wonderful chicken marsh!

29. Rice cooker Spanish chicken rice

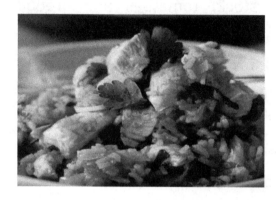

Time: 55

Serving4/5

Fixings

1) 2 tbsp. spread

2) 1 earthy colored onion (diced, medium)

3) 3 garlic cloves (cut)

4) 1 1/2 cups rice

5) 1 1/2 cups Massel Chicken Style Liquid Stock

6) 400g canned cleaved tomatoes

7) 1 tsp. ground cumin

8) 600g chicken tenderloins

9) 1/2 cup parsley (cleaved)

- Method

1.   Turn the rice cooker on to warmth and add the margarine, onion and garlic. Sauté until the onion is clear.

2.   Add the rice, stock, tomatoes and ground cumin. Lay the chicken tenderloins on top.

3.   Cover and cook for 20 mins. You may have to press the cook multiple times with a programmed rice cooker.

4.   Remove the tenderloins, cleave and get back to the pot with the hacked parsley and mix delicately to join.

30. Rice cooker quinoa porridge

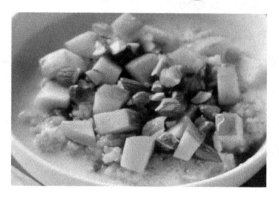

Time: 30 minutes

Serving 2/3

Fixings

1) 1/2 cup quinoa

2) 1/2 cup moved oats

3) 1 cup (250ml) water

4) 1 cup (250ml) milk (rice milk, almond milk, coconut milk are generally fine to utilize)

5) 1 medium apple, diced

6) 1/4 cup almonds, hacked

7) honey or maple syrup to shower

Strategy

1. Rinse quinoa well in a strainer under cool running water.

2.   Add to the rice cooker alongside the oats, water and milk. Spot cover on rice cooker and set the rice cooker to cook.

3.   When cooked, eliminate cover and mix (you may require some additional milk in the event that it appears to be dry).

4.   Serve into bowls and top with apples, almonds and a shower of nectar or maple syrup.

31. Rice cooker cake

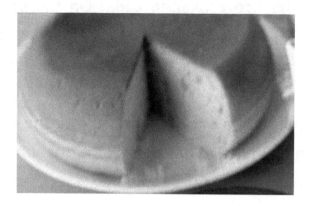

Time: 45 minutes

Serving 2/3

Fixings

    1) 2 cups self-raising flour

    2) 2 tbsp. white sugar

    3) 2 eggs (daintily beaten)

    4) 375 ml milk

Strategy

1.   Place flour, sugar and eggs into a bowl and whisk together while adding milk a little at a time until all fixings are fused.

2.   Pour cake blend into the bowl of a rice cooker and set the rice cooker to cook. On the off chance that you have a programmed rice cooker, you may have to press the traditional 2-3 times until your cake is cooked.

3.   Cook until a stick embedded into the cake tells the truth or the cake has a smooth, dry surface. This should take around 20-25 minutes.

4.   Slice and present with berries and frozen yogurt or maple syrup.

32. Rice cooker chocolate cake

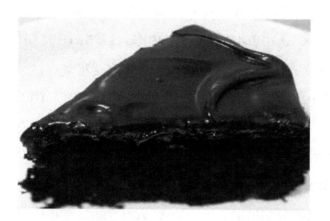

Time 45 minutes

Serving 4/5

Fixings

1) 1 cup (150g) self-raising flour, filtered

2) 1/3 cup (50g) cocoa, filtered

3) 1 cup (220g) caster sugar

4) 1/3 cup (80g) margarine, relaxed

5) 1/2 cup (125ml) milk

6) 2 eggs, softly beaten

Technique

1. Grease and flour the bowl of the rice cooker (except if it is non-stick).

2.   Place all fixings into a blending bowl and utilizing a blender, blend on high for 4 minutes or until joined.

3.   Pour combination into the rice cooker bowl.

4.   Press cook on your rice cooker. On the off chance that you have a standard rice cooker, you should press the cook button a few times until this cake is cooked. You may require a rest between each push so the temperature sensor can chill off.

5.   If you have a high level rice cooker you can pick the cake determination. Test you cake with a stick to check whether it is cooked. Turn out onto a cooling rack to cool and present with raspberries and cream.

33. Creamy Breakfast Oatmeal (Rice Cooker)

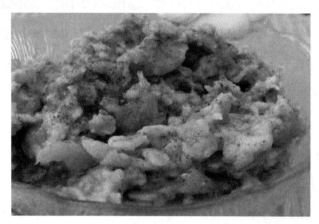

Prepared IN: 30mins

SERVES: 2

Fixings

1) 2/3 cup steel cut oats

2) 1 2/3 cups milk

3) 1 teaspoon unadulterated vanilla concentrate

4) 1 1/4 teaspoons ground cinnamon

5) 1 squeeze fine ocean salt

6) 2 tablespoons unadulterated maple syrup

7) 1/2 cup hacked dates

Bearings

1.   Place all fixings, with the exception of dates, in cooker; mix delicately to join; sprinkle dates on top.

2.   Close the cover, set on Porridge cycle.

3.   This formula is intended for a rice cooker with fluffy rationale - utilize the porridge setting. On the off chance that you have a standard rice cooker, you should watch it to decide when the cereal is done, most likely 25 to 30 minutes, contingent upon your cooker.

4.   Steel cut oats differ marginally. For certain brands I discover I need to lessen the milk to 1/2 cup to get the correct consistency.

5.   You can substitute vanilla enhanced soy milk for the milk in addition to vanilla concentrate.

34. Lemon Rice (Rice Cooker)

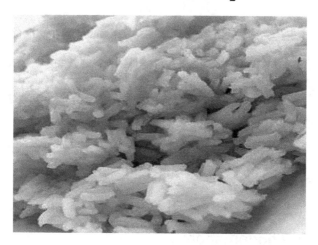

Prepared IN: 45mins

SERVES: 3-4

Fixings

1) 1 cup long grain rice

2) 1 1/2 cups chicken stock

3) 1 squeeze salt

4) 1 enormous garlic clove

5) 2 teaspoons lemon zing, newly ground

6) 2 tablespoons unsalted margarine

7) 2 tablespoons new Italian parsley

Headings

1.   Place flushed rice in the rice cooker bowl of your rice cooker.

2.   Add the chicken stock and salt; mix to join, at that point place the garlic in the middle on top of the rice.

3.   Close the cover and set for the standard cycle.

4.   When the machine changes to the Keep Warm cycle, add the lemon zing, margarine, and parsley; mix to consolidate.

5.   Close the cover and let the rice steam for 10 minutes.

6.   Fluff the rice with a wooden or plastic rice paddle or wooden spoon.

7.   This rice will hang on Keep Warm for 1-2 hours.

8.   Before serving, eliminate garlic and dispose of.

9.   Serve hot.

35. Aromatic Basmati Rice (Rice Cooker)

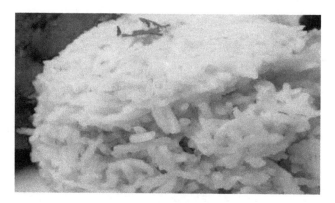

Prepared IN: 1hr 1min

SERVES: 3

Fixings

1) 1 cup basmati rice

2) 1 1/2 cups water

3) 1/4 teaspoon salt

4) 1 cinnamon stick (4 inches)

5) 3 green cardamom units

Bearings

1.   Rinse the rice in a fine sifter, at that point channel altogether.

2.   Place all fixings in the rice cooker bowl, and twirl to consolidate.

3.   Set the machine for the normal white rice cycle.

4.   When the machine movements to 'keep warm', set a clock for 15 minutes.

5.   After 15 minutes, cushion rice with the plastic oar or a wooden spoon.

6.   Serve now, or leave on 'keep warm' for as long as 4 hours.

36. Rice And Black Beans (Rice Cooker)

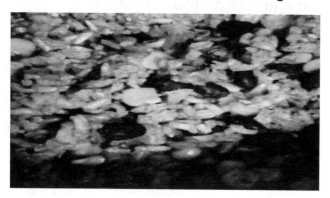

Prepared IN: 35mins

SERVES: 4

Fixings

1) 1 cup uncooked rice

2) 1 (10 ounce) can diced tomatoes with green chilies (Ro-tel)

3) 1 (14 1/2 ounce) can chicken stock

4) 1 (15 1/4 ounce) can dark beans

5) 1 (14 3/4 ounce) would sweet be able to corn (discretionary)

6) 1 cup cheddar (discretionary)

Bearings

1.   Drain tomatoes, dark beans, corn and put in Rice Cooker.

2.   Add rice, chicken stock and mix.

3.   Cook until cooker stops.

4.   Add cheddar on top.

37. Coconut Tapioca Pudding (Rice Cooker)

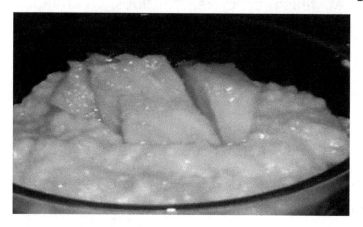

Prepared IN: 1hr 10mins

SERVES: 6

Fixings

1) 3 1/4 cups canned unsweetened coconut milk

2) 3/4 cup little pearl custard

3) 3/4 cup sugar

4) 1 enormous egg, beaten

5) 1 squeeze salt

6) 2 1/2 teaspoons unadulterated vanilla concentrate

Headings

1.   Place all fixings aside from vanilla in bowl of 6-cup rice cooker. Mix to join. Close the cover and set for Porridge cycle.

2.   Open the cover and mix momentarily like clockwork, at that point close cover.

3.   At finish of cycle, cautiously eliminate bowl from cooker. Mix in the vanilla. Fill a huge serving bowl or individual serving dishes.

4.   Let cool. Serve warm, or refrigerate covered with cling wrap.

5.   Note: little pearl custard is about the size of sesame seeds; anything bigger will take longer and require more fluid.

38. Risi E Bisi (Italian Rice And Peas) (Rice Cooker)

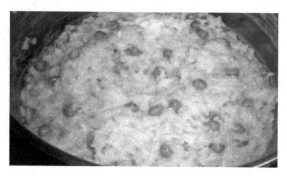

Prepared IN: 35mins

SERVES: 4-5

Fixings

1) 1 tablespoon olive oil

2) 1 tablespoon unsalted margarine

3) 1/2 cup shallot, minced (or utilize gentle onion)

4) 1/2 cup celery, minced

5) 2 tablespoons dry white wine

6) 1 cup medium-grain risotto rice (superfino Arborio, Carnaroli, or Vialone Nano)

7) 2 tablespoons medium-grain risotto rice (superfino Arborio, Carnaroli, or Vialone Nano)

8) 3 3 cups meat stock or 3 cups vegetable stock

9) 1 1/2 cups peas (new or frozen)

10)   TO FINISH

11)   2 teaspoons unsalted spread

12)   2 tablespoons hefty cream

13)   1/4 cup parmesan cheddar

Headings

1. Set Rice Cooker for the fast cook or customary cycle.

2. Place the olive oil and margarine in the rice cooker bowl.

3. When the margarine dissolves, add the shallots and celery.

4. Cook, blending a couple of times, until the shallots are relaxed yet not cooked, 2 to 3 minutes.

5. Add the wine and cook two or three minutes.

6. Add the rice and mix to cover the grains with the hot spread.

7. Cook, blending sporadically, until the grains of rice are straightforward with the exception of a white spot on every, 3-5 minutes.

8. Add the stock and peas, on the off chance that you are utilizing new, develop peas; mix to join.

9. Close the cover and reset for the Porridge cycle, or for the customary cycle and set a clock for 20 minutes.

10. When the machine changes to the Keep Warm cycle or the clock sounds, mix the rice with a wooden or plastic rice paddle or wooden spoon.

11. The rice ought to be just somewhat fluid and the rice ought to be still somewhat firm, delicate with simply bit of tooth opposition.

12. If required, cook for a couple of moments longer.

13. This rice will hang on the Keep Warm cycle for as long as 60 minutes.

14. When prepared to serve, add the peas, on the off chance that you are utilizing frozen or delicate new ones; mix just to consolidate.

15. Add the spread and close the cover or 2-3 minutes to permit to soften and the peas to warm through.

16. Stir in the cream, cheddar and salt to taste.

17. Serve right away.

39. Saffron Scented Fruity Yellow Rice - Rice Cooker

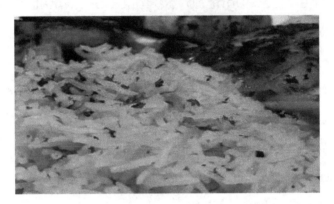

Prepared IN: 35mins

SERVES: 6

Fixings

1) 3 cups basmati rice, flushed

2) 3 cups water, to the rice cooker level

3) 1 squeeze powdered saffron (around 5 - 8 strands) or 1 squeeze saffron strand (around 5 - 8 strands)

4) 2 tablespoons organic product chutney

5) 2 - 4 cardamom cases, split and use seeds

6) salt

7) pepper

8) 1 ounce margarine

9) 2 - 4sprigs new coriander (discretionary)

Headings

1.   Important Note: This is a formula for a standard Rice Cooker - kindly change the liquids if cooking in a skillet the ordinary way.

2.   Put 3 cups 0f washed Basmati rice into your rice cooker - utilizing the cup gave.

3.   Fill up with water to the 3 cup level in the rice cooker.

4.   Add the saffron, cardamom seeds, salt, pepper and chutney to the rice and water.

5.   Using the extraordinary non-stick spatula or spoon, delicately combine everything as one.

6.   Turn the rice cooker on to the Cook cycle.

7.   (This can be kept warm when the cooking cycle has completed for as long as 2 hours.).

8.   When prepared to serve, add the margarine and delicately blend through.

9.   Then put into a serving dish or straight onto the plates and embellishment with hacked new coriander/cilantro.

10.   You can likewise sprinkle some toasted chipped almonds on top in the event that you wish.

40. Creamy Grits (Rice Cooker)

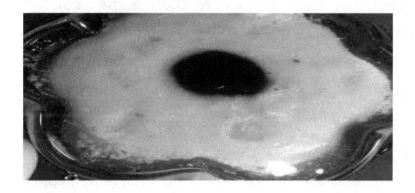

Prepared IN: 30mins

SERVES: 2

Fixings

1) 1/2 cup stone-ground corn meal

2) 1 1/2 cups milk

3) 1/4 teaspoon salt

4) 1tablespoon spread

Bearings

1.   Put all fixings into rice cooker bowl and mix to consolidate. Set to porridge cycle.

2.   About 10 minutes into the cycle, mix. (I frequently don't find time for this, and they end up fine).

3.   I present with a pat of spread and a spoonful of cherry or different jelly.

41. Greek Lemon And Dill Rice With Feta (Rice Cooker)

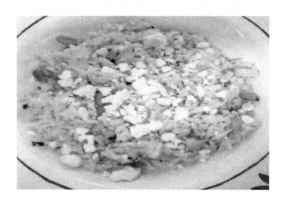

Prepared IN: 1hr 10mins

SERVES: 3-4

Fixings

1) cooking splash

2) 1 1/2 cups long grain white rice

3) 2 cups chicken stock

4) 2 tablespoons olive oil

5) 2 little bubbling onions, hacked

6) 1/4 cup pine nuts

7) 1/4 cup new lemon juice

8) 1 tablespoon minced new dill

9) 1 1/2 teaspoons minced of new mint (discretionary)

10) 1 cup disintegrated feta

11) 1 lemon, cut in 8 wedges

Bearings

1. Coat the rice bowl with cooking splash.

2. Add the rice and stock to the bowl.

3. Set the machine for the normal white rice cycle and start.

4. When the machine changes to keep warm, let it sit and steam for 10 minutes.

5. While the rice steams, heat the olive oil in a little skillet, at that point add the onions and cook for 5 minutes, mixing regularly, until delicate.

6. Add the pine nuts and cook, blending continually until they become brilliant (one moment or thereabouts).

7. When the 10 minutes of steaming are up, add the onion and pine nut combination to the rice, alongside the lemon juice, dill, and mint (if utilizing). Mix with a plastic rice paddle or a wooden spoon to join.

8. Close the cover and progress forward 'keep warm' for 10 additional minutes.

9. Transfer the rice to a serving dish, and top with the feta and lemon wedges.

42. Rice Cooker Fried Rice

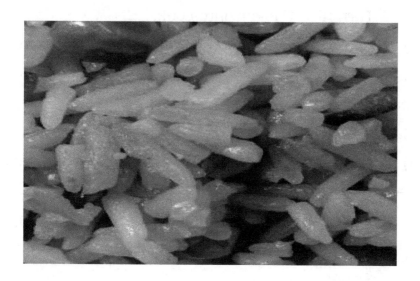

Prepared IN: 30mins

SERVES: 2-4

Fixings

1)   2 cups rice

2)   2 cups hamburger stock

3)   1 tablespoon oil (enhanced injected oil functions admirably)

4)   250 g bacon (cut into strips)

5)   1 onion (cut)

6)   1 teaspoon minced garlic

7)   1 cup frozen blended vegetables (corn parts and peas will do)

8)   2 tablespoons soy sauce

Headings

1)   Turn Rice Cooker onto cook.

2)   Add oil, bacon, onion and garlic to Rice Cooker.

3)   Stir every now and again until onion is delicate.

4)   Add rice to Rice Cooker and coat in oil.

5)   Add frozen vegetable and hamburger stock and blend well.

6)   Place top on Rice Cooker and let it do its thing.

7)   When completed blend in Soy Sauce and mix.

8)   Serve.

43. Rice Cooker Mexican Rice

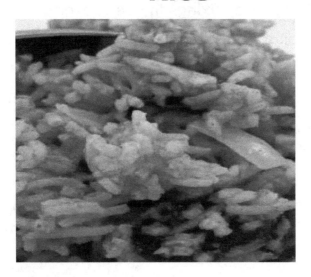

Prepared IN: 25mins

SERVES: 6

Fixings

1)   1 cup rice (I utilized long grain rice)

2)   2 1/4 cups low sodium chicken stock

3)   0.5 (6 ounce) would tomato be able to glue

4)   2 tablespoons margarine

5)   1/2 cup onion, diced little

6)   1 garlic clove, minced

7)   0.5 (4 ounce) can diced green chilies

8)   1 scramble pepper

9)   1 scramble red pepper pieces

10)   cilantro or parsley, for shading

Headings

1. Combine all fixings in rice cooker.
2. Cook as indicated by producer guidelines.
3. When cooking time completed let it sit revealed for 3 minutes or so to thicken.
4. Stir prior to serving.

44. Jamaican Grits Rice Cooker

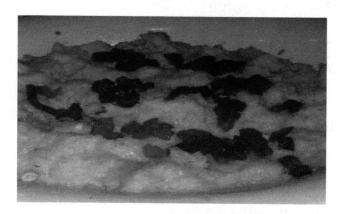

Prepared IN: 35mins

SERVES: 2

Fixings

1)   16 ounces hominy

2)   2 cups water

3)   1/2 cup corn meal

4)   1 cup cheddar

5)   1 teaspoon salt

6)   1/4 teaspoon garlic powder

7)   2 ounces pimientos

Bearings

1. Drain fluid out of hominy into estimating cup fill the rest with water until it estimates 2 cups. (Add hominy and water to rice cooker).

2. Add corn meal to water in pot (add to rice cooker start).
3. Bring to a bubble.
4. Cook.
5. When done add pimento juice and all flavors. (When done add to cooked corn meal permit to be on warm until cheddar dissolves.
6. And 1/2 cup cheddar mix.
7. Add hominy.
8. Pour in buttered dish.
9. Top with rest of cheddar.
10. Bake 350 for 25 minutes.

45. Fried Rice - Zojirushi Rice Cooker

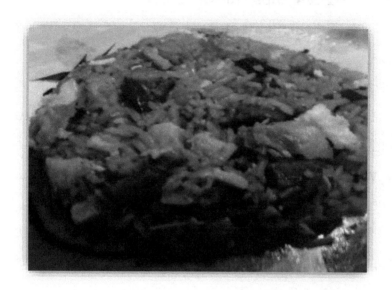

Prepared IN: 1hr 5mins

SERVES: 4-6

YIELD: 10 cups

Fixings

1. 2 cups uncooked rice
2. 1 1 cup cooked bacon or 1 cup cooked hotdog
3. 1 cup cooked chicken
4. 1 cup carrot
5. 2 eggs, mixed and hacked up
6. 1/4 cup soy sauce
7. 2 teaspoons new ginger

8. 2 teaspoons new garlic

9. 4 - 6 spring onions

10.   1 3/4 cups chicken stock

11.   2 teaspoons nut oil

12.   1/2 cup cilantro

Bearings

1)   Rinse the rice in chilly water. Change the water depending on the situation until the water is not really white. At the point when you are done, add the rice to the lower part of within the rice cooker.

2)   Mix the hotdog, chicken, carrot, soy sauce, ginger, garlic, chicken-stock, nut oil, the white piece of the spring onions. Save the green piece of the spring onions, the cilantro, and the eggs for some other time.

3)   Add the rice to the rice cooker. Pour in the blend from stage 2. Try not to MIX THE TWO. The rice will cook on the base; the blend will cook on the top.

4)   Cook the rice adhering to the rice cooker's directions. I set mine to white rice utilizing the harder cook setting (it leaves the rice a piece crunchier). It requires around 40 minutes with my rice cooker.

5)   When the rice is finished cooking, add the remainder of the spring onions, the cilantro, and the cooked eggs. Mix the rice to blend the fixings and close the top. Leave it in the "warm" setting for 10 minutes.

6)   Enjoy!

46. Turkey Barley Goulash Casserole (Rice Cooker)

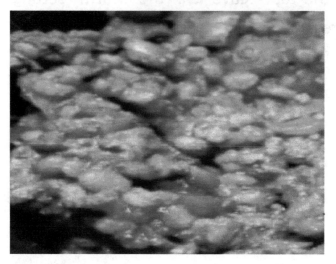

Prepared IN: 45mins

SERVES: 4

Fixings

1) 1 lb. lean ground turkey or 1 lb. ground hamburger

2) 1/2 cup hacked onion

3) 1/4 cup hacked celery

4) 1 red chime pepper, diced

5) 1 carrot, destroyed

6) 3/4 cup grain

7) 1 (6 ounce) would tomato be able to glue

8) 1 1/2 cups water

9) 1 1/2 teaspoons salt

10)   1/4 teaspoon pepper

11)   1 garlic clove, minced

12)   1 tablespoon Worcestershire sauce (discretionary)

13)   2 tablespoons red wine (discretionary)

14)   2 teaspoons sweet paprika (discretionary)

Bearings

1)   Set rice cooker to "Speedy Cook" or on the off chance that you don't have that setting simply turn on the rice cooker. Throw in initial five fixings, shutting cover in the middle cleaving to keep the warmth inside. Look like clockwork and mix to separate turkey bunches, at that point close the cover once more.

2)   When turkey is cooked, add rest of fixings. In the event that you don't have the last three flavors, you can forget about them or substitute your own top picks.

3)   Close cover and set rice cooker to brown rice setting. In the event that you don't have an earthy colored rice setting, set it for white rice. At the point when it completes, check to guarantee grain is cooked through. On the off chance that grain is still too chewy, let it run another cycle. It should require around 40 minutes. On the off chance that blend is excessively dry, add somewhat more water.

5)   Top with cheddar or parmesan cheddar on the off chance that you wish.

Conclusion

I would like to thank you for choosing this book. It contains recipes which are healthy and can easily be made in the rice cooker. Hope these will help you in making dishes easily using a rice cooker. Prepare at home and appreciate along with your family members.

 I wish you all good luck!